Walking by Faith and Not by Sight with Stage 3 Breast Cancer

by

Cornice Brown

Dedication

My dedication to God in this book helped me to write it. With God's help, I can do all things through Christ who strengthens me. But most important it was the love of God. For God so loved the world (John 3:16). This helped motivate me in my faith walk, to help others who needed encouragement with the battle of cancer or any kind of disease. To all Cancer Survivors and Believers of Jesus Christ, Trust in the Lord (Proverbs 3:5-6).

Acknowledgment

My knowledge is to tell the true story of my faith walk, being a Native of Charleston SC (the holy city), a daughter, a mother, a wife (divorced), sister, aunt, niece, cousin, friend, a prayer warrior, neighbor, co-worker and a believer of Jesus Christ, knowing that the things which are impossible with men are impossible with God (Luke 18:27). Read this faith book and believe in your heart, because in 2017, until present, God did it and is continuing doing it for Cornice Simmons Brown.

I'm a survivor of Stage 3 Breast Cancer.

Table of Contents

"Loving God has always been something I have been taught since I was a child growing up in the church. Even though that taught me to believe in Him, it was something different. So, at the age of 51, I had to walk by faith and not by sight. It was either trust God or die! This book will allow me to tell my story about my faith in God. A true faith walk with Jesus Christ!"

Chapter 1

Believing was a choice for me, but having faith was a demand because, without faith, it is impossible to please God. (Hebrews 11:6). It started in late November 2016. I had a vision of a man with an all-white jacket, like a doctor. He told me if I didn't drink water for thirty days, I would die. At that time, I became afraid. It was mostly fear, but I knew that I had to do what the vision said because I trusted God in everything: my walk and my ways. So, I started fasting. I drank water for thirty days, and I ate one meal a day. I knew that God Almighty wanted my attention, and something was about to happen. I started seeking His face and will for my life by fasting, praying, and reading the word of God (The Holy Bible), the King James version. I attended prayer services and Bible study. I would arrive early so I could lay on the altar and cry out to Him because Cornice Brown needed to die so His spirit could work within me. Everything about me took off the old and put on the new. I accepted Christ when my daughter was four (in 1987); she's 33. I still had some bad things about me that needed to die. Every generational curse, every evil and wicked thought, feeling, and emotion needed to die so God could live more in me. So I drank water (no other drink) but ate one meal a day for thirty days plus the entire month of December, January, and February. I was still praying and fasting, laying before him. Around the month of April, I found a lump in my left breast, so I started to make arrangements to go visit my primary doctor. He set up a mammogram appointment. I went to have it done in the month of May and they saw the lump was the size of a golf ball. I kept my faith and trusted God because God had prepared me for this battle. The nurses became very emotional, but I kept my cool because I believed in the Almighty power of God. I declared Isaiah 53:5 and Isaiah 54:17. I went to a breast specialist in June (the day my son was graduating from high school). I was diagnosed with stage 3 Breast Cancer in the year of 2017.

Chapter 2

My journey began. I told my Apostle about everything when it first started. She began to laugh and stated the devil doesn't know who he is messing with. You got this. She began to fast for me because my journey needed spiritual strength as well as physical strength. I began to ask God: Why me? He began to speak to me. I could hear Him clearly, and He quoted, "So that I could get the glory out of it." My healing will deserve more praise and His honor. Thanks to God, people would be able to see my healing and would give God the glory, honor, and praise because it all belongs to Him. I began to read the story of the three Hebrew boys, Daniels 3:16-18 They were put in the fiery furnace because they refused to bow down to their king as a god. I refused to bow down to cancer and any benefits of it because Jesus died so that I could live and not die, declaring the work of God for my life. I started chemotherapy on July 31, 2017. They told me the good and bad about it, but I kept the faith, and I walked by faith and not by sight. (2 Corinthians 5:7). I was supposed to have eight treatments every second Monday, but I heard God speak to me, and He gave me instructions. He told me to anoint my daughter's hands because she would care for me, and the day before chemo, I walked around the building three times(father, son, and holy ghost). I remembered that Joshua walked around the wall of Jericho for seven days. (Joshua:6). I followed my instructions the day before I walked around the building praying for the doctor, nurses, patients, and assistants. I declared and decreed the power of the three anointing of God to send the healing

Angels. When I got to the fourth treatment, the doctor said, "That's enough treatment." I was supposed to have eight treatments, but God knew that I only needed four because chemo is very strong; it destroys good cells and bad cells. I was walking by faith and not by sight. They could not see, but I could! I did get weak through this journey, but I heard God speak and said I have not left you nor forsaken you. (Deuteronomy 31:6 &Hebrew 13:5). I remembered this lump was the size of a golf ball, and with only four treatments, it shrank to nothing. The treatment from God dissolved it. This was faith. I had to be put in the fire like the Hebrew boys to know who He (God) really was. He is God. They suggested that I remove both breasts. I had a double mastectomy on 11/15/2017. God is good and worthy to be praised. Through this journey, I needed protection from the enemy. The spirit of God told me to anoint my daughter's hands because she was the one to care for me and protect me physically. The angels of the Lord were always with me, but I needed natural protection because the battle was a warfare battle. My daughter made sure I ate the food that was good for my body. She did everything the doctors required me to do, but I kept in tune with God about everything, even medication, and my surroundings.

Chapter 3

During my chemo, I was still capable of working. God gave me strength from day to day. I made sure my schedule was converted for my faith journey. God took care of my financial needs. After surgery on 11/17, I knew that His healing angels were always present. I kept praying, declaring, and decreeing Isaiah 53 & Isaiah 54 over my life. Psalms 23 was my favorite scripture. My grandmother, the late Mrs. Lucille Simmons, always told me that I needed to know that the Lord is my shepherd. During this faith walk, I lost my hair, but I didn't lose my faith in God. Sometimes, it was unbearable, but I kept remembering Isaiah 53, But He was wounded for our transgressions, He was bruised for our iniquities: the chastisement of our peace was upon him; and with his stripes, we are healed. I kept declaring Psalms 17:8. I also reminded the Almighty God that You said in Deuteronomy 31:6-8 that You would not leave me nor forsake me. This was when my faith was at its lowest point. This is when I kept quoting scriptures. I played it on the phone so the enemy could understand that Jeremiah 29:11, for I know the plans for you declares the Lord. I continued to cry out to Him every day, listening to God, Gospel music, praise, and worship. Because the battle with cancer was not mine; the Lord, only God, brought me through it. Cornice's flesh wanted to give up the day they told me I had stage 3 Breast Cancer, but God said I can do all things through Christ who strengthens me (Philippians 4:13). I needed the strength to get through, so I began to walk by faith and not by sight (2 Corinthians 5:7). I could not see it but I believed it from the bottom of my soul. God also gave me songs that helped me. “This is my story. This is my song, praising my Savior all day long. He knows my name.” Knowing that God knew my name made my radiation therapy (4-6 weeks of radiation) go smoothly. This radiation is meant to kill the cells left behind. They had to be destroyed, even though God kept me in perfect peace Isaiah 26:3.

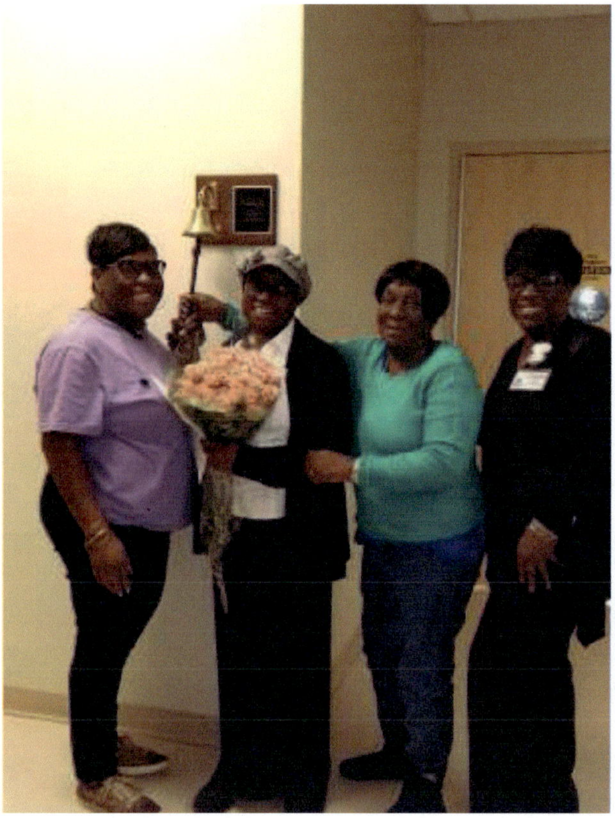

left Lolita Simmons (daughter) , me center,

(Cornice Brown) , Susie M. Brown (aunt)

And Lanell Simmons (sister) family love matters

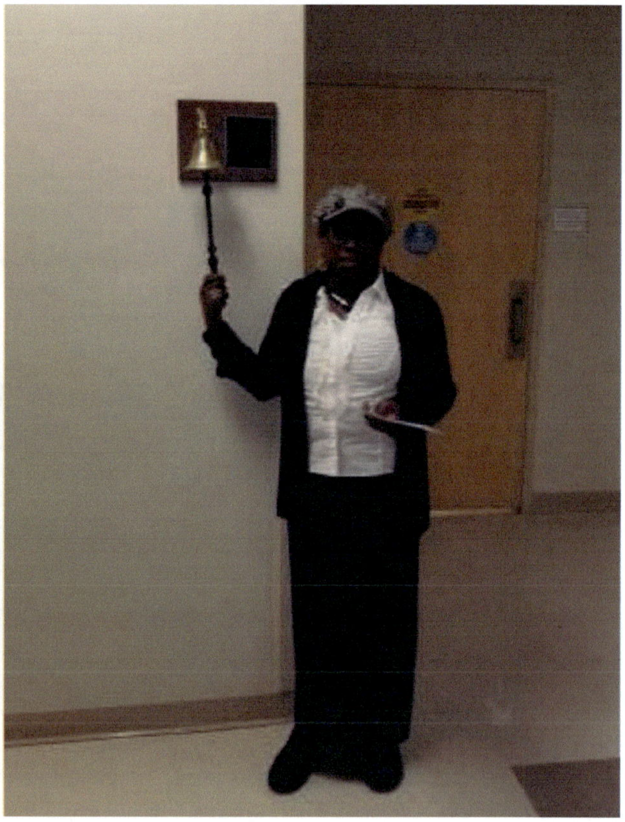

Rang the bell; February 7,2018

Chapter 4

How could I believe in someone I had never seen? If I could trust the doctors, then I knew I could trust the Almighty God because the only option I had was to die. So, I began to study the word of God. You did it for the three Hebrew boys, Daniel:3; they were put in the fiery furnace because they refused to bow down to the king as a god. So I said I'm not bowing down to Stage 3 Breast Cancer; I'm going to bow down to my Almighty God. That was my faith. I began to trust Him because if He did it for them, He could do it for me. I began to thank Him for my healing every day, even when it wasn't. I knew it was something I needed to do because cancer was here only for a season! The story of Solomon 1 King 3:4-5 because I knew that I needed to do more. I thought about Solomon. He sowed, and God showed up that same night and asked him what he wanted, so I said, "God, I don't have what Solomon had, but what do I have to do to get through?" The spirit of God told me what, and I began to sow from that time until now for my healing because my seed is my faith. If I pay my bills, I get to keep everything flowing in the natural, but in the spiritual rim, I keep my healing flowing. The manifest of His Glory can continue to move my life. I can live a long life like the Bible said, so sowing was a great part of my life. So, sowing was a great part of my faith walk. I planted my seed for healing, and I watered it while continuing to sow for my healing. My praise is my worship, and my worship was fertilizer for my seed to grow. When praises go up, blessings come down. I need the blessings of God to come down for me.

Chapter 5

Now, faith is the substance of things hope for, the evidence of things not seen Hebrews 11:1, I could not see it, but I believed in God's word. I kept declaring my healing and thanking God for total healing, yes I did have a little doubt when the chemo got overbearing, but I called on the strong saints of God who could encourage me to give me the strength to call on the Almighty God (Jesus Christ) The physical part wanted to give up but my spiritual part kept reminding me who is the almighty God Jesus Christ my Savior. The Lord is my light and my salvation. Whom shall I fear? Psalm 27:1 I could not fear cancer because the Lord is the strength of my life of whom shall I be afraid. I knew deep inside that God was always with me because the holy spirit kept reminding me that He promised never to leave me or forsake me Hebrew13:5. This journey was so God could get the glory out of it, meaning that I had to work in faith to receive and operate in the glory and faith work by love (Galatians 5:16). The love I had for God was more than anything I prayed and asked him to replace my love with agape love of God because on this journey I knew I had to love everybody, even my enemies. For God so loved the world that He gave His only begotten son John 3:16. That love was greater than any man can ever imagine. I remember that after my surgery, an emergency was out of town, and I was asked to go to the situation. It was hard, but I knew it was an assignment because when I got there, it was difficult. But I called on the saint of God, my prayer warriors, and my Apostle. I knew that God wanted me to go because one morning, listening to the

5:30 a.m. prayer line just as clear as a phone call, I heard my Apostle's voice now faith Hebrew 11:1. All I could do was worship the Lord because I was in Ohio. She was in South Carolina, but that's how God works. He is amazing. God is awesome in all His ways. He is the same today, yesterday, and forever more (Hebrews 13:8). If He did it in the Old Testament and the New Testament of the Holy Bible, He can do it for me in 2017-2018 and present. Remembering when I told my Apostle about my stage 3 breast cancer, she began to laugh. The devil doesn't know who he's messing with. You got this because God has you. I always believed and trusted in God, but when cancer came, it was like speaking to my mountain (Isaiah 54:10). Taking on the love of the Almighty God, I had to kill Cornice in order to walk in faith in everything about me. I had to take off the old way of thinking and put on the new way of God Romans 12:2. I had to be transformed (Cornice Brown) in order to be healed. I changed my surroundings because faith in God is really up to you. If you can believe in things in the world that will let you down by making promises they cannot keep instead of believing in the king of kings, lord of lords. He's a doctor in the sick room, a lawyer in the courtroom, and my financial advisor, my banker, my heart fixer, and my mind regulator. He did it for the children of Israel, the three Hebrew boys. He healed the sick and raised the dead. He healed my body from stage 3 breast cancer, and this is all faith. I believed and trusted in the word of God (Bible) from Genesis to Revelations, for the promises of God are secured. This faith walk was personal because it made me a better person (woman) to depend on the Almighty power of God to trust Him in His word.

Chapter 6

Love covers a multitude of sinful faults (1 Peter 4:17 and 2 Corinthians 5:7). Walking by faith and not by sight, you must walk in love. Love your enemies as you love yourself. Love everyone because God is love. For God so loved the whole world that He gave His only begotten son (John 3:16). Report daily asking God the known and unknown to forgive you of your sins (Matthew 6:9-13). The Lord's prayer is the best that I do daily in the morning, at noon, and at bedtime (any time of the day). I needed God to do something in my life. Cornice Brown needed healing from the Almighty God, so I needed to do everything that the word of God required me to get. I needed to humble myself to the Almighty God. I needed to walk in love and repentance of myself because I needed to walk in the spirit of God, but I needed to humble myself into the spiritual rim of God in order to be healed. Knowing that only God can do it, I begin to seek ye first the kingdom of God (Matthew 6:33).

Chapter 7

Without faith, it is impossible to please God (Hebrews 11:6). I need to trust God because He is Alpha, Omega, and Almighty God, but why? Why not my oncology doctor, the nurses, and the medication? Society tells us to trust them, but God works through these natural things to prove the spiritual things in our lives. I had to trust God. Having faith to believe that I wanted to please Him by praying, fasting, sowing, and worshiping Him. Giving God thanks for my healing by declaring and decreeing the word of God. When He created the Earth, it was faith He spoke, and it formed. I believed it, and it was done. My job was to please God by being ordained to Him, keeping His commandments, and believing the impossible for my healing, restoring, and renewing of my body, mind, and spirit. God told me that I had to go through it so that He could get the glory. The glory is the transformation of my body, the total healing of my entire body, walking in the glory of the all mighty God Jesus Christ telling others with cancer and other diseases that you must please God Jesus Christ the Almighty Savior because if you can't please him, your faith walk is going to be long and hard but if you stay attuned with him weeping may endure for a night but joy will come in the morning Psalm 30:5. God loves His children but we must endure pain and suffering but if we trust him and have faith we can endure.

Chapter 8

(James 2:26) Faith without works is dead. Faith must be worked by you. You have to have faith in yourself to say I can do all things through Christ. (Philippians 4:13) I remember having a dream that I was flying over South Carolina, and when I got to Ashley River, I began to walk on the water. I know that with faith, I could conquer cancer because I remember the story of Peter (Matthew 14:28-29). Then, I knew if I kept my eyes on Jesus Christ, that I could do this. I worked on my faith by knowing that the dream was my faith walk, that I could walk on water if I continued to trust in Jesus Christ; that my cancer walk was like Peter walking on water. It was time I took my eyes off Jesus, but Ashley River could not hold me down because Jesus Christ had His eyes on me, and I had my eyes on Him. Jesus is so amazing because it was that time when I was feeling low, but I began to give Him praise and glory, for He has been so good to me, better than I was to myself. I would begin to praise him as David did - for my healing. This was the time I just had chemo. I just gave him praise because when praises go up, blessings come down. I will praise the name of God with a song, Psalm 69:30. When I begin to lift my hands, the Glory of God begins to surround me, and I cry out with thanksgiving. The Angels of Glory began to fill the room. My healing angels were always with me. I call my angels forward every day, morning, noon, evening, and midnight. My angels of protection and prosperity were always with me.

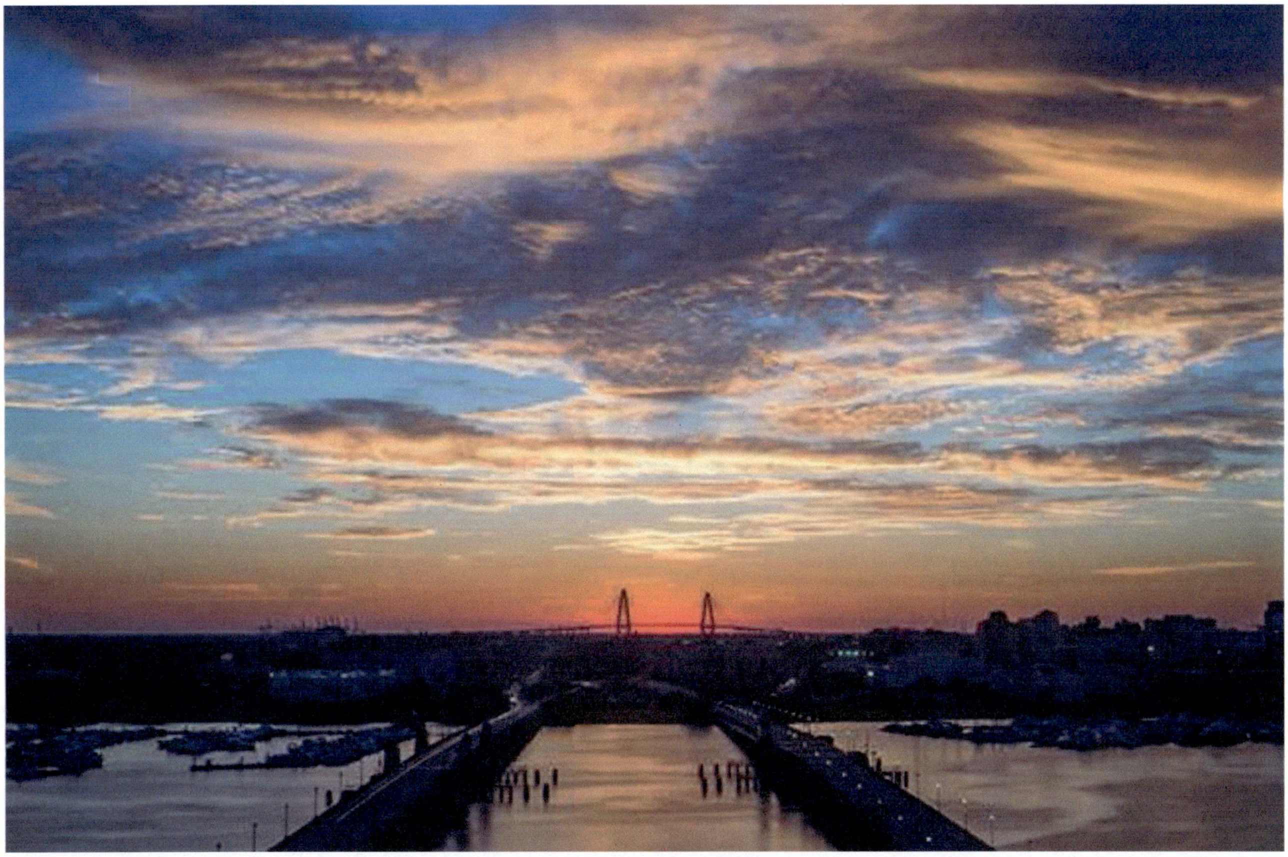

(Charleston, SC, Ashley River Bridges)

Chapter 9

The operation of my faith walk was when the doctor said that your numbers are excellent with cancer. The doctor goes by your blood count. When you get to the oncology doctor, they draw your blood, and the level of your blood count determines if you have cancer or not. My numbers have always been at the rate it should be. From 2018 to 2022, I learned how to walk by faith and not by sight. It's now 2022, five years of being cancer-free (Thank the Lord). I take it one day at a time. I continue to believe and never doubt. If I doubt, I repent, asking God to forgive (repent). Sometimes, the process takes long but to keep the faith, you cannot see it, but you must believe it in your heart. Everyone around you may talk and not believe, but you must believe and declare the works of God (Jesus Christ) for your life. Always remember that life and death are in the power of your tongue (Proverbs 18:21). Speak good things about your life and the generation to come. God promised Abraham and Sarah a son (Genesis 17) in their old age, and that promise was fulfilled. It took years, but the promises of God are certain (Jeremiah 29:11). He knew the plans for my life, and all I had to do was walk in them. The manifest of His glory for my life was the healing of Stage 3 Breast Cancer. During my journey, I had a vision that I was driving over the Ravenel Bridge, and when I got to the end, there were tolls, but Charleston doesn't have tolls. My body was ejected from the car. I began to fly in the air, and when I saw my car, it had already come through the toll and made it to the other side of the bridge. My revelation of this dream was that Jesus already paid the price when He died for me and took the beating for me (Isaiah 53:3-12). All I needed was to believe and walk in the total healing of God for my life.

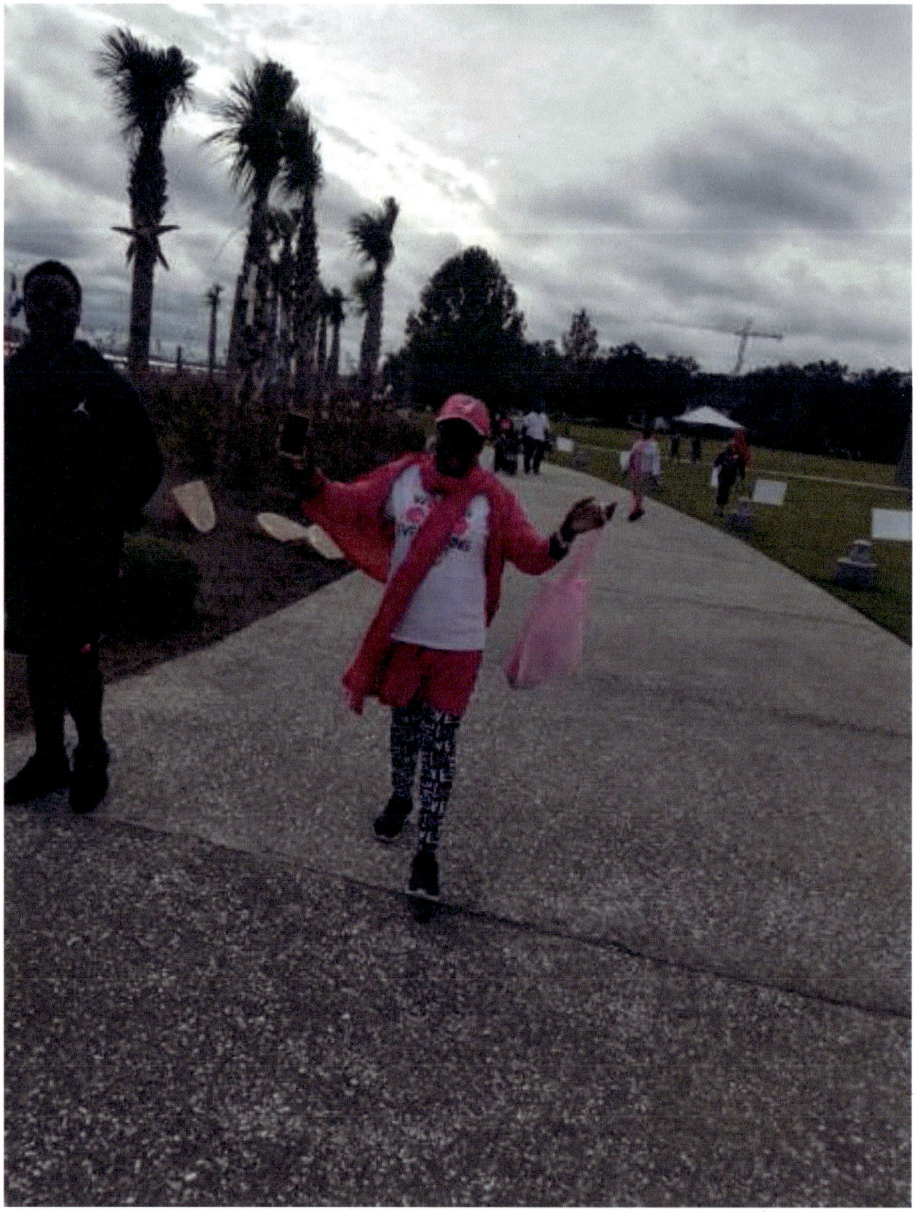

Victory Walk at the American Cancer Society on October 27, 2017

Conclusion

There is nothing too hard for God; what He did for Cornice Brown, He can do for you (the entire world). Jesus Christ provided for me my entire life (56 years). When situations in your life seem to weigh you down, walk by faith and not by sight (2 Corinthians 55:7). Believe in Jesus Christ, who created the heavens and Earth. Do not weaver but trust in the Lord with all your heart (Proverbs 3:5-6). Lean not to your own understanding in all your ways. Acknowledge Him, and He will direct your path.

Love,

Cornice Brown

Cancer Survivor

Summary

Love and forgiveness was also a major part in my walk. Love covers a multitude of sins. (1 Peter 4:8).

So I started telling everyone, "I Love you always" and meant it from my heart because God so loved the world that He give His only begotten son (John 3:16) so I had to give Him my all mind, heart, body, spirit and my seed (sowing).

When I began doing this, everyone began to love me more (taking off the old & walking in the new me). Having a support team was also very important - someone to lean on to help you continue in the faith. My faith-believing team was always near: my sister Lanell Simmons, my Dad (who's now deceased), my daughter Lolita T. Simmons, my son Gary D. Brown Jr. , my aunties, uncles, cousins, my husband (now ex-husband) and his family, my spiritual mother, my Apostle and Church family, co-workers, especially the pharmacy, and all my friends American Cancer Society.

This is what made my faith walk: Walking in love, Keeping God's first commandment. (Matthew 22:37)

Made in the USA
Monee, IL
05 November 2026

67382286R00017